Unwrapping the Allergy Mystery

The Truth Behind Christmas Tree Allergies

By

Shirley L. Brooks

Table of content

Introduction

 The Christmas season is a period of euphoria, festivity, and harmony. For some, one of the most loved customs is designing a Christmas tree, occupying the room with the fragrance of pine and shimmering lights. However, allergies may be an unwelcome guest at this festive tradition for some people.

In this article, named "Opening Up the Sensitivity Secret: Reality Behind Christmas Tree Sensitivities," we will dive into the universe of Christmas tree sensitivities and reveal reality behind this normal yet frequently got peculiarity wrong. By grasping the causes, side effects, and executives of Christmas tree sensitivities, we desire to assist you and your friends and family in partaking in a safe and sensitivity-free Christmas season.

Allergies to Christmas trees Allergies to Christmas trees are allergic reactions to allergens that are present in or near Christmas trees. Although it is commonly held that tree pollen is to blame for these allergies, the truth is more nuanced. Different allergens, like shape spores, dust bugs, and tree sap, can set off hypersensitive responses in vulnerable people.

Sensitivities happen when the insusceptible framework blows up to a substance that is commonly innocuous, regarding it as a danger. When exposed to allergens, people with sensitivities might encounter a range of side effects, including wheezing, hacking, irritated eyes, blockage, and skin rashes. In extreme cases, sensitivities can prompt more serious responses, for example, trouble breathing or hypersensitivity.

For those who suffer from allergies or have loved ones who do, it is essential to understand the causes of allergies to Christmas trees and how to manage them. We want to provide you with the knowledge and tools to make informed decisions about Christmas tree selection, decoration, and maintenance so that everyone can have a happy and allergy-free holiday season by deciphering the mystery of these allergies.

Understanding and overseeing allergies during the Christmas season is of extreme significance because of multiple factors:

1. Wellbeing and Prosperity: A person's health and well-being can be significantly impacted by allergies. It can be difficult to fully enjoy the holiday festivities if you suffer from symptoms like sneezing, coughing, and itchy eyes. By getting it and overseeing sensitivities, people can limit their side effects and keep up with great wellbeing during this unique season.

2. Quality Time with Friends and Family: The Christmas season is a period for social events with loved ones. Notwithstanding, assuming somebody in the family experiences sensitivities, their side effects can hose the delight and keep them from completely taking part in exercises. By successfully overseeing sensitivities, people can guarantee that they can invest quality energy with their friends and family without the weight of awkward side effects.

3. Safety: For people with extreme sensitivities, openness to specific allergens can present serious wellbeing risks. Anaphylactic responses, which can be dangerous, are a worry for certain people with sensitivities. By getting it and overseeing sensitivities, people can play it safe to stay away from possible allergens and guard themselves during the Christmas season.

4. Inward feeling of harmony: anxiety and stress can be brought on by allergies, especially around the holidays when allergens may be more common. By understanding the triggers and going to proactive lengths to oversee sensitivities, people can enjoy harmony of psyche, realizing that they have done all that could be within reach to limit their openness to allergens and decrease the risk of hypersensitive responses.

5. Delight in Customs: On many occasions, customs, for example, beautifying a Christmas tree or baking merry treats, can accidentally expose people to allergens. People can continue to participate in these cherished activities without jeopardizing their health by becoming

aware of the specific allergens associated with these customs and putting in place the appropriate strategies.

All in all, understanding and overseeing sensitivities during the Christmas season is critical for keeping up with great wellbeing, appreciating quality time with friends and family, guaranteeing security, discovering a sense of psyche reconciliation, and completely partaking in valued customs. By doing whatever it takes to forestall and oversee sensitivities, people can have a cheerful and sensitivity-free Christmas season.

Chapter 1: Understanding Allergies

Understanding sensitivities is fundamental for actually overseeing and alleviating their effect on our wellbeing. To assist you in comprehending the concept of allergies, here are a few key points:

1. Definition: Sensitivities are strange, resistant reactions to substances that are regularly innocuous to a great many people. These substances, which are referred to as allergens, can take a variety of forms, including pollen, dust mites, pet dander, certain foods, medications, insect venom, and a variety of other things.
2. Response of the Immune System: At the point when an individual with sensitivities comes into contact with an allergen, their resistant framework erroneously distinguishes it as a danger. Accordingly, the resistant framework discharges synthetics, for example, receptors, which trigger a range of hypersensitive side effects.
3. Unfavorably susceptible Responses: Depending on the individual and the allergen, allergic reactions can manifest in a variety of ways. Sneezing, coughing, itching, watery eyes, skin rashes, hives, and more severe reactions like anaphylaxis and difficulty breathing are all common symptoms.
4. Allergen Sharpening: Over time, allergies can develop. At first, openness to an allergen may not bring about any observable responses. Nevertheless, rehashed openness can sharpen the resistant framework, prompting the improvement of unfavorably susceptible side effects upon resulting experiences with the allergen.
5. Sensitivity Types: Food allergies, skin allergies (such as eczema and contact dermatitis), drug allergies, and insect allergies are just a few examples of the many types of allergies. Specific symptoms and triggers are unique to each type.
6. Sensitivity Testing and Conclusion: On the off chance that you suspect you have sensitivities, counseling an allergist or immunologist for appropriate testing and

diagnosis is significant. Skin pricks or blood allergy tests, for example, can help determine which allergens are causing your symptoms.

7. Treatment and Management: Sensitivities can be overseen through a blend of evasion measures, medicine, and immunotherapy. Common management strategies include avoiding allergens, taking antihistamines or nasal sprays, and carrying an auto-injector of epinephrine for severe allergies. Over time, immunotherapy, like allergy shots or sublingual tablets, can help the immune system become less sensitive.

Individuals can make informed decisions to reduce their exposure to allergens, seek appropriate treatment, and lead a healthier and more comfortable life by comprehending the underlying mechanisms and triggers of allergies.

Common allergens

Common allergens include:

1. Pollen: Dust from trees, grasses, and weeds is a typical allergen, prompting sensitivities to pollen or roughage fever.
2. Dust vermin: These minuscule organisms can cause allergic reactions and can be found in upholstery, bedding, and dust in the home.
3. Pet dander: Aversions to pet dander, which incorporates skin pieces, spit, and pee, are normal among people who are delicate to creatures.
4. Form spores: Form can fill in clammy conditions, like washrooms, cellars, and regions with water harm, and its spores can cause hypersensitive responses.
5. Bug toxin: Stings or nibbles from bugs like honey bees, wasps, hornets, and fire insects can prompt unfavorably susceptible responses in certain people.
6. Foods: Peanuts, tree nuts, milk, eggs, wheat, soy, fish, and shellfish are all common food allergens. The

symptoms of these allergies can range from mild to severe.
7. Medications: Certain prescriptions, like anti-microbials (e.g., penicillin), nonsteroidal calming drugs (e.g., headache medicine), and a few sedatives, can set off hypersensitive responses in vulnerable people.
8. Latex: People who are exposed to natural rubber latex-based products like gloves, balloons, and medical devices can develop a latex allergy.

It is essential to keep in mind that these are only a few examples of common allergens; numerous other substances can trigger allergic reactions in various individuals. Distinguishing explicit allergens through testing and talking with a medical services expert is vital for legitimate findings and the board of sensitivities.

How allergies develop and why some people are more prone to allergies

Sensitivities arise when the insusceptible framework overcompensates for innocuous substances (allergens) like dust, pet dander, or certain food sources. Hereditary variables assume a part, making certain individuals more inclined to sensitivities. Moreover, natural elements, early openness to allergens, and a family background of sensitivities can contribute to expanded helplessness.

1. Genetics: family background of sensitivities increases helplessness.

2. Invulnerable Framework Responsiveness: A few people have invulnerable frameworks that blow up ordinarily innocuous substances.

3. Ecological Elements: Openness to poisons, smoke, or certain synthetic substances can contribute to sensitivity advancement.

4. Exposures during infancy: The absence of early openness to different organisms might influence invulnerable framework advancement, expanding sensitivity risk.

5. Hypothesis of Hygiene: A weaker immune system and increased susceptibility to allergies may result from being raised in overly clean environments.

6. Physical Location: Living in regions with high dust counts or explicit allergens can hoist the gamble of creating sensitivities.

7. Dietary Impacts: The development of allergies may be affected if particular foods or dietary factors are introduced early.

8. Feelings of anxiety: Ongoing pressure might impact the safe framework, possibly expanding weakness into sensitivities.

9. Polluting the Air: Openness to elevated degrees of air contamination has been connected to an expanded gamble of sensitivities.

Keep in mind that these elements frequently interact, making the interaction between the environment and genetics complex.

Different kinds of allergic reactions

The types and severity of allergic reactions can vary. Normal sorts include:

1. Reactions to the skin: like hives, skin inflammation, or dermatitis.

2. Reactions to the airways, like shortness of breath, wheezing, sneezing, or coughing.
3. Eye responses: conjunctivitis or eye itchiness
4. Gastrointestinal responses: queasiness, spewing, or looseness of the bowels.
5. Anaphylaxis is a serious, life-threatening reaction that can affect multiple systems. It can cause a drop in blood pressure, make it hard to breathe, and make you lose consciousness.

Recognizing allergens and looking for clinical guidance for legitimate management is significant. Unfavorably susceptible responses can appear in different ways. It's critical to take note of the fact that these various kinds of unfavorably susceptible responses can change in their seriousness and treatment choices. For proper diagnosis and treatment, it is best to consult a healthcare professional if you suspect you have an allergic reaction.

Chapter 2: Christmas Tree Allergies: Fact or Fiction?

Allergies to Christmas trees do exist. Although not all people are allergic to Christmas trees, some people may be sensitive to tree pollen, Mold spores, or other allergens from live or artificial Christmas trees. Here are a few vital elements to consider:

1. Live Christmas trees: Certain individuals might be susceptible to tree dust, which can be delivered by live Christmas trees. Sneezing, coughing, itchy eyes, and a runny nose are all signs of this.

2. Spores of mold: Live Christmas trees can hold onto spores, particularly in the event that they are kept in a clammy climate. These spores have the potential to be released into the air when brought inside, resulting in allergic reactions in those who are susceptible.

3. Tree sap and sap: The sap or gum from live trees might cause skin aggravations or contact dermatitis in touchy people, bringing about redness, irritation, or rashes.

4. fabricated trees: While counterfeit Christmas trees don't create dust or have shape spores, they can gather dust, which can set off sensitivities in certain people. If the tree is stored in an area with a lot of dust, dust mites may also be a problem.

Here are some suggestions to reduce allergies caused by Christmas trees:

- Think about a fake tree, assuming you have known aversions to tree dust or shape.

- On the off chance that you select a live tree, shake it completely to eliminate free dust and potential spores prior to bringing it inside.
- Keep live trees all around watered to prevent them from drying out, which can deliver more allergenic particles.
- Think about involving an air purifier or keeping the tree in a very well-ventilated region to decrease allergen fixation.
- It is best to get personalized advice and preventative measures from a healthcare professional if you have severe allergies or asthma.

Eventually, Christmas tree sensitivities are not fiction, but rather the probability and seriousness of hypersensitive responses will shift among people.

Debunking common myths about Christmas tree allergies

1. Myth: Christmas Trees Cause Allergies.

Reality: True Christmas tree allergies are uncommon, despite the fact that real trees can contain pollen and mold spores. Unfavorably susceptible responses are almost certain because of residue or form on put-away counterfeit trees.

2. Myth: Pine tree allergies.

    Reality: Pine tree allergies are uncommon. Mold spores, dust, or pollen from the tree may be the source of the majority of reactions.

3. Myth: Just genuine trees trigger allergies.

    Reality: Counterfeit trees can collect residue and form while away, causing unfavorably susceptible responses. Cleaning on a regular basis can help reduce this risk.

4. Myth: Allergic reactions always occur right away.

    Reality: Over time, allergies can manifest. If symptoms appear after decorating, think about other things in the environment that could be to blame.

5. Myth: Everything is resolved by removing tree allergens.

    Reality: Indoor allergens like residue and pet dander can, in any case, cause responses. Guarantee great indoor air quality to decrease, generally speaking, the sensitivity risk.

6. Myth: Everyone has the same reaction.

    Reality: Allergies fluctuate among people. What causes one person to react may not affect another.

7. Myth: Every fake tree has no allergies.

    Reality: Counterfeit trees can assemble residue and shape, particularly whenever put away in sodden circumstances. Prior to use, proper cleaning is essential.

Keep in mind that if you think you might be allergic, you should see an allergist for a precise diagnosis and tailored guidance.

Identifying the real culprits behind allergic reactions during the holiday season

1. Dust Parasites:

    Culprit: dust collected on enhancements, materials, and put-away things.

    Prevention: routine maintenance, particularly in storage areas.

2. Spores of mold:

   Culprit: Present on genuine Christmas trees, put away adornments, or in sodden indoor spaces.

   Prevention: Keep improvements dry, clean consistently, and think about counterfeit trees.

3. Pet Dander:

   Culprit: carpets, furniture, and guest-brought pet allergens.

   Prevention: Utilize air purifiers, vacuum frequently, and create pet-free areas.

4. Pollen:

   Culprit: bringing outdoor items inside, live wreaths, or decorations.

   Prevention: Shake off open-air items and think about counterfeit embellishments.

5. Fragrances:

   Culprit: Scented candles, blends, or deodorizers.

   Prevention: Select unscented options and open windows for ventilation.

6. Allergens to Food:

   Culprit: occasional feasts containing normal allergens.

Prevention: Obviously name dishes, convey sensitivities, and deal sans allergen choices.

7. Smoke:

Culprit: chimney smoke, candles, or incense.

Prevention: Guarantee appropriate ventilation and use options like electric candles.

Recognizing and limiting openness to these guilty parties can assist with decreasing the risk of hypersensitive responses during the Christmas season. For individualized guidance, see an allergist if symptoms persist.

Differentiating between tree-pollen allergies and other tree-related allergies

Most of the time, allergies to tree pollen are caused by pollen that trees release into the air during their reproductive cycle. Sneezing, a stuffy or runny nose, and itchy eyes are some of the symptoms. Other tree-related sensitivities might include contact with tree rind, sap, or leaves, prompting skin aggravation or unfavorably susceptible dermatitis. An allergist can assist with distinguishing explicit triggers through testing and give fitting administration systems.

Tree Dust Sensitivities:

Culprit: airborne dust delivered by trees for propagation.

Season: Ordinarily tops in spring when trees discharge a lot of dust.

Symptoms: fatigue, itchy or watery eyes, runny or stuffy nose, and sneezing

Triggers: a wide range of trees, including oak, birch, cedar, and pine, depending on the kind of pollen.

Tree pollen allergies are specifically referred to as allergies brought on by tree pollen. This kind of sensitivity is set off when people come into contact with the dust grains delivered by unambiguous tree species. Sneezing, a runny or stuffy nose, itchy or watery eyes, coughing, and fatigue are all signs of tree pollen allergies. The typical season for these allergies is spring, when trees release their pollen.

However, the term "other tree-related allergies" can also be used to describe reactions to other tree parts, such as the bark, leaves, or sap. These sensitivities might appear as skin rashes, tingling, hives, or even respiratory side effects like hacking or wheezing. Other tree-related allergies, in contrast to allergies to tree pollen, can occur at any time of the year and are not always seasonal.

It is vital to take note that tree dust sensitivities are a particular kind of sensitivity brought about by the dust grains delivered by trees, while other tree-related sensitivities can be brought about by different parts of trees, not simply dust.

Differentiating between tree pollen allergies and other allergies related to trees can be made easier with an understanding of the specific triggers, symptoms, and timing. If you're not sure, talking to an allergist can help clarify things.

Chapter 3: Allergens Associated with Christmas Trees

Christmas trees can convey allergens that might set off responses in certain people. These allergens can include:

1. Spores of mold: Christmas trees, particularly in the event that they're live and have been cut for some time, can hold onto spores. When brought inside, these spores might be delivered very high, possibly causing respiratory issues.

2. Dust: Dust can build up on artificial trees that have been stored for a long time, which could be a problem for people who have allergies to dust.

3. Pesticides: Live trees might be treated with pesticides, and deposits could represent a gamble for those sensitive to these synthetic compounds.

4. Tree sap: Handling live trees can expose people to tree sap, which can sometimes irritate the skin or cause allergic reactions.

5. Pollen: Despite the fact that Christmas trees are ordinarily not significant dust sources, certain individuals might, in any case, be delicate to the dust on the tree.

To limit the gamble, consider completely cleaning counterfeit trees before use and deciding on newly cut trees if picking a live one. Moreover, permitting the tree to ventilate in a carport or comparative space prior to bringing it inside can assist with lessening possible allergens. It is best to get personalized advice from an allergist if a person has known allergies.

How these allergens can trigger allergic reactions

Allergens related to Christmas trees can set off hypersensitive responses through different instruments:

1. Inhalation: When the tree is handled or decorated, dust and mold spores may escape into the air. People might breathe in these particles, prompting respiratory side effects like sniffling, hacking, and trouble relaxing.

2. Skin to Skin: Tree sap or buildups from pesticides on live trees can come into contact with the skin. Sensitive individuals may experience redness, irritation, or an allergic reaction as a result of this contact.

3. Exposed Mucous Membrane: Sap or pollen can get in the eyes if you handle a Christmas tree, especially a live one. Itching, redness, and watery eyes may result from this.

4. Ingestion: Even though it is less common, children, in particular, run the risk of having allergens transferred from their hands to their mouths. This can occur on the off chance that hands come into contact with allergenic substances on the tree and contact the face or mouth.

Individual reactions change, and certain individuals might be more sensitive to these allergens than others. Individuals with known sensitivities or respiratory circumstances ought to be wary while dealing with Christmas trees and think about going to preventive lengths, like wearing gloves, cleaning the tree prior to bringing it inside, and guaranteeing great ventilation in the home. It is essential to seek medical attention right away if a person experience severe allergic reactions.

Identifying potential sources of allergens in Christmas trees

Potential sources of allergens in Christmas trees include:

1. Shape Spores: Live trees, particularly whenever cut and put away for some time, may hold onto shape spores. These spores have the potential to spread through the air and cause allergic reactions if brought inside.
2. Mold and dust on fake trees: In the event that fake trees are put away for quite a while, they can collect residue and shape. Additionally, dust mites may be present, which can exacerbate allergic reactions.
3. Pesticides: Live Christmas trees might be treated with pesticides to forestall bugs. Leftover pesticides can represent a gamble for people sensitive to these synthetic substances.
4. Tree sap: Dealing with live trees can expose people to tree sap. Sap on hands or the tree can irritate the skin and cause allergic dermatitis.
5. Pollen: Live trees can produce pollen, but they are not a major source. Individuals sensitive to tree dust might encounter respiratory side effects.
6. Contagious Allergens: Notwithstanding mold spores, parasites present in the tree or its current circumstances can be allergenic.

Consider cleaning artificial trees prior to use, inspecting live trees for signs of mold or pests, and allowing live trees to air out before bringing them indoors to reduce the number of allergens that are exposed. It's best to get personalized advice from an allergist if someone already knows they have allergies.

Chapter 4: Managing Christmas Tree Allergies

To oversee Christmas tree sensitivities:

1. Pick the Right Tree: Choose a fake tree in the event that residue or form sensitivities are a worry. In the event that you are picking a live tree, go for a newly sliced one to limit shape development.

2. Examine the Tree: Really take a look at live trees for indications of shape, bothers, or noticeable residue. Before bringing the tree inside, shake it outside to get rid of any loose allergens.

3. Clean Fake Trees: Wipe down and clean counterfeit trees to eliminate dust that might have gathered during stockpiling.

4. Ventilate: Increment ventilation in the home by utilizing fans or opening windows to diminish indoor allergen levels.

5. Gloves and Handwashing: Wear gloves while taking care of the tree to limit skin contact with expected allergens. Wash hands completely subsequent to embellishing.

6. Limit Openness: Limit time spent around the tree, particularly for people with known sensitivities. Consider utilizing air purifiers to assist with diminishing airborne allergens.

7. Quickly Remove the Tree: In order to avoid prolonged exposure to potential allergens, if you use a live tree, you should think about removing it from the house right after the holidays.

8. Counsel an Allergist: On the off chance that sensitivities endure or deteriorate, counsel an allergist for testing and customized exhortation on overseeing side effects.

By making these strides, you can partake in the Christmas season while limiting the risk of setting off hypersensitive responses related to Christmas trees.

Prevention measures to minimize exposure to allergens

To limit openness to allergens, consider the accompanying counteraction measures:

1. fabricated trees: Pick a fake tree to stay away from potential allergens like form, dust, and sap related to live trees.

2. Investigate Live Trees: On the off chance that you are choosing a live tree, investigate it for indications of shape, bothers, or noticeable residue. Shake the tree outside to eliminate any free allergens prior to bringing it inside.

3. Clean Fake Trees: Wipe down and clean fake trees prior to enlivening to eliminate gathered dust.

4. Ventilation: Increment ventilation in your home by utilizing fans or opening windows to lessen indoor allergen levels.

5. Handwashing and Gloves: Wear gloves while taking care of the tree to limit skin contact with likely allergens. After decorating, thoroughly wash your hands.

6. Air Purifiers: Use air purifiers with HEPA channels to assist with eliminating airborne allergens.

7. Limit Openness Time: Avoid spending too much time near the tree, especially if you know someone who has allergies. In order to concentrate allergens in a single location, designate specific areas for tree decorating.

8. Immediate Tree Removal: In the event that you are utilizing a live tree, eliminate it immediately after the Christmas season to forestall delayed exposure to expected allergens.

9. See an allergist: Consult an allergist for individualized advice on managing symptoms and testing if allergies persist or get worse.

By carrying out these avoidance measures, you can partake in the Christmas season while diminishing the risk of allergen openness.

Choosing the right type of tree to reduce allergy risks

Consider the following suggestions when selecting a Christmas tree:

1. Choose trees with females: Female trees produce less dust than male trees. Choosing a female tree can help reduce exposure because pollen can be a common allergen.

2. Pick Low-Dust Assortments: It is generally believed that some tree varieties, like fir, spruce, and pine, produce less pollen.

3. Examine Live Trees: In the event that you are picking a live tree, review it for shape, bugs, or indications of rot prior to buying. Shake the tree to eliminate free trash.

4. Clean Artificial Trees: Before installing artificial trees, clean them to get rid of any dust or allergens that may have accumulated during storage.

5. Use Allergen-Lessening Designs: Pick hypoallergenic or non-allergenic enhancements to limit expected triggers.

6. Ventilate the Inside: Guarantee great ventilation while embellishing by opening windows to diminish indoor allergen levels.

7. Counsel an Allergist: On the off chance that sensitivities are a huge concern, talk with an allergist for customized exhortation and potential sensitivity testing.

8. Fake Trees: Choose a fake tree to kill the gamble of form, dust, and sap related to live trees. If the tree is going to be kept for a long time, make sure it is clean and free of dust.

9. Fir or Tidy Trees: Consider varieties of fir or spruce when selecting a live tree. These trees are more averse to creating a lot of dust compared with other tree types.

10. Trees Just Cut: To keep mold at bay, select a live tree that has just been cut down. More established trees put away in sodden circumstances might have higher spore counts.

11. Examine the Tree: Before purchasing live trees, thoroughly inspect them for signs of mold, pests, or dust. To remove any stray particles, shake the tree outside.

12. Think about pruned trees: pruned trees can be a decent choice, as they are less inclined to hold onto shape spores. Guarantee that the fertilized soil is liberated from toxins.

13. Sensitivity Amicable Tree Choices: If you don't want to use a live or artificial tree, you can still create a festive atmosphere by using smaller, decorated branches or unconventional materials.

At last, individual inclinations and explicit sensitivities ought to direct your decision. On the off chance that somebody in your family has known sensitivities, talking with an allergist can give customized guidance on choosing a tree that limits potential allergen openness.

Proper tree maintenance and cleaning techniques

Techniques for proper tree care and cleaning for both live and artificial Christmas trees can help reduce allergens and ensure a healthier holiday atmosphere

For live trees:

1. Assess the Tree: Live trees should be examined for signs of mold, pests, or dust prior to purchase. Pick a newly sliced tree to limit its development.

2. Shake the outside: Before bringing the tree inside, shake it outside to get rid of any loose needles, dust, or other potential allergens.

3. Water and Trim: Trim the tree's trunk prior to putting it in water to further develop water retention. Keep the tree stand loaded up with water to keep it from drying out and shedding more allergens.

4. Ventilate: Increment ventilation in the room where the tree is set to lessen indoor allergen levels.

5. Breath Expulsion: Eliminate the tree quickly after the Christmas season to forestall delayed openness to expected allergens.

For artificial trees:

1. Clean and inspect: Prior to beautifying, assess counterfeit trees for residue and garbage. Wipe down the tree with a soggy fabric or utilize a vacuum cleaner with a brush connection to eliminate dust.

2. Storage: Store fake trees in a dry, cool spot to prevent shape development. To keep it safe while being stored, think about using a tree storage bag.

3. Handwashing and Gloves: Wear gloves while taking care of a counterfeit tree to limit skin contact with residue and allergens. Wash hands completely in the wake of enrichment.

General Tips:

1. Employ HEPA Filters: Use a HEPA-filtering air purifier if you have an artificial tree to help reduce allergens in the air.

2. Designated Place for Decorating: To limit allergens to a single space, concentrate tree decorating in one area.

You can enjoy a festive atmosphere while minimizing the potential allergen exposure associated with Christmas trees by following these

Chapter 5: Alternative Decorations for Allergy Sufferers

Alternate decorations that won't exacerbate allergy symptoms can be used to create a festive atmosphere for allergy sufferers

1. Texture and Strip Style: Use texture and lace to make bows, festoons, and different designs that don't create residue or allergens.
2. Non-allergenic decorations: pick adornments produced using materials like glass, metal, or plastic rather than conventional materials that might set off sensitivities.
3. Counterfeit Plant Life: In the event that live plants are a worry, decide on counterfeit vegetation like wreaths and laurels produced using sensitive cordial materials.
4. Driven Lights: To reduce the accumulation of dust and allergens, opt for LED lights rather than standard incandescent ones. Driven lights are likewise more energy-productive.
5. Elective Tree Choices:

   - Wooden Trees: Consider a wooden or texture-covered tree elective.
   - Wall Decals: If you don't have any actual decorations, you can still create a festive atmosphere with holiday-themed wall stickers or decals.

6. Fragrance-Free Candles: Stay away from scented candles, as the aromas can set off sensitivities. Settle on unscented candles or flameless Drove candles.
7. Texture Tree Skirt: Rather than a live tree, utilize a texture tree skirt to add a beautifying touch without the potential allergens associated with genuine trees.
8. Ornaments made by hand: Utilize allergy-friendly materials like felt, fabric, or non-allergenic clay to create personalized ornaments.
9. Pinecone Options: Consider decorative alternatives like wooden or fabric pinecone replicas if pinecones irritate your allergies.
10. Pillows and throws for the season: Improve your home's merry feel with occasional cushions and tosses produced using hypoallergenic materials.

When decorating, choose items that are less likely to cause allergic reactions and be mindful of the materials used. For allergy sufferers, regular dusting and cleaning of decorations can also contribute to a healthier indoor environment.

Exploring alternative options to traditional Christmas trees

Consider these elective choices for customary Christmas trees for an exceptional and well-disposed occasion stylistic theme:

1. Wooden Tree: Make a wooden tree construction or wall decoration, enhanced with lights and trimmings.

2. Bed Christmas Tree: Make a rustic and adaptable alternative to the traditional Christmas tree by repurposing wooden pallets.

3. Tree of Branch: Gather beautiful branches or utilize an exposed tree limb to form a moderate and regular tree elective.

4. String Light Tree: String lights can be used to draw a tree shape on a wall to create a glowing, space-saving decoration.

5. Tree on chalkboard: Draw or stencil a Christmas tree on a blackboard wall or board and enhance it with chalk decorations.

6. Sculpture of a Metallic Tree: Choose a tree-shaped sculpture made of metal or wire with ornaments.

7. Hanging Decorations: Suspend an assortment of balancing decorations at different lengths to frame a merry occasion.

8. Quill or Sparkle Tree: For a contemporary and allergy-friendly alternative, construct a tree out of feathers or metallic tinsel.

9. Paper Tree: Make a paper tree utilizing collapsed or sliced-out paper to make an outwardly engaging and lightweight enrichment.

10. Texture Tree: Use texture or felt to make a delicate and contact-cordial tree elective, reasonable for those with responsive qualities.

11. Evergreen Wall Decals: Apply evergreen tree decals to a wall for a bubbly look without the use of regular materials.

These choices give a scope of innovative choices for occasion improvements, guaranteeing a lively climate while obliging sensitivity concerns

Allergy-friendly decorations and ornaments

Select sensitivity-agreeable enhancements and decorations that limit expected triggers. Here are a few ideas

1. Hypoallergenic Trimmings: Pick trimmings produced using materials like glass, metal, or plastic rather than regular materials that might hold onto allergens.

2. Texture Trimmings: Pick texture-based adornments, for example, felt or fabric, which are more averse to setting off sensitivities.

3. Non-Scented Style: Stay away from scented adornments or designs to forestall hypersensitive responses set off by aromas.

4. Garlands and artificial wreaths: To avoid potential allergens, choose artificial wreaths and garlands made of hypoallergenic materials.

5. Luminous LEDs: Utilize drone lights rather than customary lights to keep away from potential respiratory aggravations related to consuming candles.

6. Decor in Metallic: Pick metallic or non-permeable designs that are not difficult to perfect and are more averse to holding onto allergens.

7. Paper Stylistic Theme: Consider paper-based embellishments like origami or cut-out snowflakes for a bubbly look without allergen concerns.

8. Wooden Style: To reduce the likelihood of coming into contact with mold or other allergens, choose decorations made of sealed or treated wood.

9. Tree Skirt Free of Allergens: Select a tree skirt produced using hypoallergenic materials, keeping away from textures that might trap residue or allergens.

10. DIY Clay Decorations: Make your own decorations utilizing sensitivity-aware materials like air-dry mud.

11. Launderable Improvements: Select decorations that are simple to clean, such as items that can be washed or wiped.

Make sure to clean embellishments before use, store them in dry circumstances, and be aware of any known allergens in materials. Along these lines, you can create a merry environment without settling for less sensitive concerns.

Creative ways to celebrate the holiday season without a real tree

Commend the Christmas season innovatively without a genuine tree with these elective thoughts:

1. Do-It-Yourself Decoration Show: On a decorative stand or branches in a vase, put festive ornaments on display.

2. Wall-Mounted Tree: Use string lights or washi tape to make a tree shape on a wall, then, at that point, enhance with trimmings.

3. On the Wall, a Felt Tree: Cut a tree shape from brilliant felt and connect it to a wall. For a child-friendly option, use felt ornaments as decorations.

4. Book Stack: For a literary and decorative touch, stack books with holiday themes in the shape of trees.

5. Hanging Trimming Versatile: Make a portable utilizing a series of trimmings, making an interesting and eye-getting occasion improvement.

6. Pruned Plant Stylistic Theme: Improve pruned plants with merry lights and trimmings to bring a bit of occasion soul inside.

7. DIY Glitter: Use paper, fabric, or felt to make your own garland to decorate walls or mantels.

8. Decor for the Windows: Hang merry window sticks, paper patterns, or pixie lights to make an occasion scene.

9. Occasion Focal point: orchestrate occasional things like pinecones, candles, and trimmings in a brightening highlight.

10. A Tree of Twigs Accumulate twigs or branches and arrange them in a jar or pot. Enrich with little trimmings or lights.

11. String Lights Party: Hang string lights in imaginative examples or shapes, carrying a warm and happy vibe to your space.

12. Display from Winter Wonderland: Enrich a tabletop with counterfeit snow, smaller than expected winter-themed dolls, and Drove candles.

Keep in mind that special times of year are tied to creating a warm and euphoric environment. Enjoy the holiday season in a manner that satisfies your preferences and takes into account any allergies you may have by being imaginative and customizing your decorations.

Chapter 6: Seeking Professional Help

Looking for proficient assistance prior to picking a Christmas tree may not be a typical practice, but you can unquestionably avoid potential risks to guarantee a safe and sensitive, well-disposed decision.

1. Get advice from an allergist. Assuming you have explicit worries about tree-related sensitivities, consider talking with an allergist. They can perform tests to recognize likely allergens and give customized exhortations.

2. Research Tree Assortments: Investigate tree assortments known to be less allergenic, like fir or tidy. A horticulturist or allergist might be able to tell you which trees are less likely to cause allergies.

3. Consideration of Artificial Trees: Use an artificial tree if you're worried about natural allergens. To prevent mold growth, make sure it has been stored in dry conditions.

4. Examine Live Trees: Check a live tree for visible decay, mold, or insects before purchasing it. To remove any loose materials, shake the tree.

5. Pick Female Trees: Female trees regularly produce less dust than male trees. On the off chance that dust is a worry, choose a female tree.

6. Ventilation: While bringing the tree inside, guarantee great ventilation to limit exposure to any allergens present.

7. Clean Fake Trees: Before putting up artificial trees and decorations, wipe down any dust or other potential allergens.

8. Take into consideration allergen-friendly decor. Choose ornaments and decorations that are hypoallergenic and made of less allergenic materials.

Keep in mind that even though taking these steps can help lower the risk of having an allergic reaction, it is always a good idea to get professional help if you have specific health issues or allergies that you are aware of. Talking with an allergist or horticulturist can give you a custom-fit direction in light of your unique conditions.

When to counsel an allergist or immunologist

Counseling an allergist or immunologist is fitting in different circumstances, including:

1. Sensitivity side effects: On the off chance that you experience steady or extreme sensitivity side effects like wheezing, tingling, hives, or respiratory issues.

2. Repetitive Sinus Contaminations: In the event that you have continuous sinus contaminations or constant sinusitis, sensitivities can be a contributing element.

3. Asthma Concerns: Assuming you have asthma and suspect that sensitivities might be setting off or fueling your side effects.

4. Skin problems: if you have allergic skin conditions like eczema or dermatitis.

5. Food Sensitivities: On account of thought or affirmed food sensitivities, particularly in the event that you experience extreme responses (hypersensitivity).

6. Bug Sting Sensitivities: Assuming that you have had extreme responses to bug stings, an allergist can survey the situation and suggest suitable measures.

7. Allergies to Medicines: An allergist can help you find alternatives if you suspect or have allergies to medications.

8. Word-related sensitivities: if you think the environment in your workplace causes allergic reactions.

9. Immunodeficiency Concerns: If you have frequent or severe infections, this may point to an immunodeficiency underneath.

10. Quality of Life Implications of Allergies: If allergies have a significant impact on your quality of life, activities of daily living, and sleep.

11. Unknown Symptoms: for unexplained or repetitive side effects that might be connected with sensitivities or insusceptible framework problems.

An allergist or immunologist is prepared to analyze and deal with a great many hypersensitive and immunologic circumstances. In the event that you have worries about your wellbeing and suspect sensitivities or safe framework issues, talking with an expert can give you important bits of knowledge and assist with making a fitting administration plan.

Allergy testing and diagnosis

Allergy testing and diagnosis ordinarily include the following advances:

1. Clinical History: Your symptoms, as well as their frequency and duration, and any potential triggers, will be inquired about during the allergist's initial examination of your medical history.

2. Actual Assessment: An actual assessment might be conducted to assess the presence of any noticeable, unfavorably susceptible responses or related side effects.

3. Conversation of Triggers: Talk about unambiguous triggers or conditions where you experience side effects, helping guide the testing and handling.

4. Sorts of Sensitivity Testing: Sensitivity testing should be possible through different techniques:

Skin Prick Test: Limited quantities of allergens are applied to the skin using a little needle.

A blood test (RAST or ImmunoCAP) responds to allergens by measuring specific antibodies (IgE).

Patch Check: Applied to the skin to identify allergies to contact, particularly eczema and dermatitis.

5. Interpreting the Findings: Results are ordinarily accessible not long after the tests. Positive outcomes demonstrate aversions to explicit allergens.

6. Challenge testing (if necessary): At times, challenge testing might be conducted, where the patient is exposed to possible allergens in a controlled environment under clinical watch.

7. Findings and Treatment Plan: The allergist will make a diagnosis and talk about the best options for treatment based on the results of the tests and the clinical evaluation.

8. Aversion to Allergens: Direction on staying away from distinguished allergens in day-to-day existence to limit openness and side effects.

9. Management of medications: Remedy or non-prescription drugs might be prescribed to oversee side effects.

10. Immunotherapy (sensitivity shots): To gradually desensitize the immune system, allergen immunotherapy (allergy shots) may be suggested for some allergies.

It's essential to take note that sensitivity testing ought to be directed under the management of a certified allergist. Inaccuracies may result from self-diagnosis or reliance solely on online resources. In the event that you suspect sensitivities, talk with a medical professional proficient in legitimate testing and direction custom-fitting to your particular circumstance.

Treatment options for managing Christmas tree allergies

To oversee Christmas tree sensitivities, think about the accompanying treatment choices:

1. Antihistamines: Over-the-counter allergy medicines can assist with mitigating side effects like sniffling, tingling, and a runny or stodgy nose brought about by openness to tree allergens.
2. Nasal Decongestants: Decongestant nasal showers or oral decongestants might give alleviation from nasal clogs, yet drawn-out utilization of nasal splashes ought to be kept away from to forestall bounce-back blockage.
3. Nasal Sprays of Corticosteroids: Sprays that can be purchased over-the-counter or prescribed can help alleviate allergy symptoms by reducing inflammation in the nasal passages.

4. Eye Drops: For those encountering bothersome or aggravated eyes, over-the-counter or remedy eye drops can provide alleviation.

5. Sensitivity Shots (Immunotherapy): In order to gradually de-sensitize the immune system, allergens are injected into the body in small amounts through allergy shots. Talk with an allergist to examine in the event that this is a reasonable choice.

6. Strategies for Avoidance: Limit openness to allergens by picking elective embellishments, selecting counterfeit trees, or completely cleaning and ventilating live trees prior to bringing them inside.

7. Air Purifiers: Use air purifiers furnished with HEPA channels to assist with eliminating airborne allergens from the indoor climate.

8. Proper upkeep of trees: In the event that you are utilizing a live tree, do whatever it takes to limit allergens by shaking it outside, routinely watering it, and speedily eliminating it after the Christmas season.

9. Talk with an allergist: In the event that side effects endure or deteriorate, look for direction from an allergist. They are able to carry out tests to locate specific allergens and offer suggestions for the best treatments.

It's crucial to tailor the methodology in view of individual side effects and inclinations. Always seek individual guidance and treatment options from a medical professional.

Conclusion

Understanding the potential allergens associated with live and artificial Christmas trees reveals the truth about allergies to these trees. Shape spores, dust, and different variables can contribute to unfavorably susceptible responses during the Christmas season. While some people may be more susceptible to allergies, taking preventative measures like selecting hypoallergenic trees, maintaining them appropriately, and controlling the environment can help reduce risks.

During the Christmas season, elevated familiarity with expected allergens and their sources is essential. People with realized sensitivities ought to find proactive ways to limit openness, and talking with an allergist can give important bits of knowledge. By picking sensitive cordial beautifications, appropriately keeping up with trees, and executing preventive measures, people can establish a merry climate while focusing on their wellbeing and prosperity. In general, allergy management and awareness contribute to a healthy holiday celebration.

Encouraging readers to enjoy a safe and allergy-free Christmas

As you get ready to commend the happy season, let the delight of special times of year be joined by a pledge to a safe and sensitivity-free Christmas. Here are a few uplifting statements:

1. Pick Shrewdly: Pursue informed decisions while choosing Christmas trees, considering hypoallergenic choices, and reviewing live trees for expected allergens.

2. Deck the corridors Carefully decorate your space with care and enjoyment. Pick-sensitivity amicable trimmings and enrichments produced using non-allergenic materials.

3. Ventilate and Clean: Guarantee great ventilation during enlivening to diminish indoor allergen focuses. Clean the area around the tree on a regular basis to keep dust and allergens from building up.

4. Individualized Methods of Prevention: Make your needs the focus of preventative measures. Consult an allergist for tailored guidance and testing if allergies are a concern.

5. Accumulate Knowledge: Spread mindfulness among loved ones about potential allergens related to Christmas trees, empowering everybody to establish a protected climate.

6. Focus on Wellbeing: Make your health and wellbeing a priority. If you are aware that you have allergies, take precautions to limit your exposure, and seek professional help if your symptoms persist.

7. Respectful Celebration: Make choices that are in line with your health goals and contribute to a joyful, allergy-free celebration as you responsibly enjoy the festivities.

Keep in mind that the Christmas season is a period of happiness, warmth, and harmony. By integrating sensitivity and mindfulness into your festivals, you can guarantee a protected and sound Christmas for you as well as your friends and family. I wish you a festive season filled with joy, laughter, and precious moments.